General view of the agriculture of the county of Nairn, the eastern coast of Inverness-shire, and the parish of Dyke, and part of Edenkeillie, in the county of Elgin, and Forres

James Donaldson

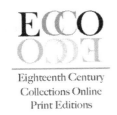

Eighteenth Century
Collections Online
Print Editions

Gale ECCO Print Editions

Relive history with *Eighteenth Century Collections Online*, now available in print for the independent historian and collector. This series includes the most significant English-language and foreign-language works printed in Great Britain during the eighteenth century, and is organized in seven different subject areas including literature and language; medicine, science, and technology; and religion and philosophy. The collection also includes thousands of important works from the Americas.

The eighteenth century has been called "The Age of Enlightenment." It was a period of rapid advance in print culture and publishing, in world exploration, and in the rapid growth of science and technology – all of which had a profound impact on the political and cultural landscape. At the end of the century the American Revolution, French Revolution and Industrial Revolution, perhaps three of the most significant events in modern history, set in motion developments that eventually dominated world political, economic, and social life.

In a groundbreaking effort, Gale initiated a revolution of its own: digitization of epic proportions to preserve these invaluable works in the largest online archive of its kind. Contributions from major world libraries constitute over 175,000 original printed works. Scanned images of the actual pages, rather than transcriptions, recreate the works *as they first appeared.*

Now for the first time, these high-quality digital scans of original works are available via print-on-demand, making them readily accessible to libraries, students, independent scholars, and readers of all ages.

For our initial release we have created seven robust collections to form one the world's most comprehensive catalogs of 18th century works.

Initial Gale ECCO Print Editions collections include:

History and Geography
Rich in titles on English life and social history, this collection spans the world as it was known to eighteenth-century historians and explorers. Titles include a wealth of travel accounts and diaries, histories of nations from throughout the world, and maps and charts of a world that was still being discovered. Students of the War of American Independence will find fascinating accounts from the British side of conflict.

Social Science

Delve into what it was like to live during the eighteenth century by reading the first-hand accounts of everyday people, including city dwellers and farmers, businessmen and bankers, artisans and merchants, artists and their patrons, politicians and their constituents. Original texts make the American, French, and Industrial revolutions vividly contemporary.

Medicine, Science and Technology

Medical theory and practice of the 1700s developed rapidly, as is evidenced by the extensive collection, which includes descriptions of diseases, their conditions, and treatments. Books on science and technology, agriculture, military technology, natural philosophy, even cookbooks, are all contained here.

Literature and Language

Western literary study flows out of eighteenth-century works by Alexander Pope, Daniel Defoe, Henry Fielding, Frances Burney, Denis Diderot, Johann Gottfried Herder, Johann Wolfgang von Goethe, and others. Experience the birth of the modern novel, or compare the development of language using dictionaries and grammar discourses.

Religion and Philosophy

The Age of Enlightenment profoundly enriched religious and philosophical understanding and continues to influence present-day thinking. Works collected here include masterpieces by David Hume, Immanuel Kant, and Jean-Jacques Rousseau, as well as religious sermons and moral debates on the issues of the day, such as the slave trade. The Age of Reason saw conflict between Protestantism and Catholicism transformed into one between faith and logic -- a debate that continues in the twenty-first century.

Law and Reference

This collection reveals the history of English common law and Empire law in a vastly changing world of British expansion. Dominating the legal field is the *Commentaries of the Law of England* by Sir William Blackstone, which first appeared in 1765. Reference works such as almanacs and catalogues continue to educate us by revealing the day-to-day workings of society.

Fine Arts

The eighteenth-century fascination with Greek and Roman antiquity followed the systematic excavation of the ruins at Pompeii and Herculaneum in southern Italy; and after 1750 a neoclassical style dominated all artistic fields. The titles here trace developments in mostly English-language works on painting, sculpture, architecture, music, theater, and other disciplines. Instructional works on musical instruments, catalogs of art objects, comic operas, and more are also included.

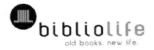

The BiblioLife Network

This project was made possible in part by the BiblioLife Network (BLN), a project aimed at addressing some of the huge challenges facing book preservationists around the world. The BLN includes libraries, library networks, archives, subject matter experts, online communities and library service providers. We believe every book ever published should be available as a high-quality print reproduction; printed on-demand anywhere in the world. This insures the ongoing accessibility of the content and helps generate sustainable revenue for the libraries and organizations that work to preserve these important materials.

The following book is in the "public domain" and represents an authentic reproduction of the text as printed by the original publisher. While we have attempted to accurately maintain the integrity of the original work, there are sometimes problems with the original work or the micro-film from which the books were digitized. This can result in minor errors in reproduction. Possible imperfections include missing and blurred pages, poor pictures, markings and other reproduction issues beyond our control. Because this work is culturally important, we have made it available as part of our commitment to protecting, preserving, and promoting the world's literature.

GUIDE TO FOLD-OUTS MAPS and OVERSIZED IMAGES

The book you are reading was digitized from microfilm captured over the past thirty to forty years. Years after the creation of the original microfilm, the book was converted to digital files and made available in an online database.

In an online database, page images do not need to conform to the size restrictions found in a printed book. When converting these images back into a printed bound book, the page sizes are standardized in ways that maintain the detail of the original. For large images, such as fold-out maps, the original page image is split into two or more pages

Guidelines used to determine how to split the page image follows:

• Some images are split vertically; large images require vertical and horizontal splits.
• For horizontal splits, the content is split left to right.
• For vertical splits, the content is split from top to bottom.
• For both vertical and horizontal splits, the image is processed from top left to bottom right.

GENLRAL VIEW

OF THE

GRICULTURE

OF THE

JNTY OF NAIRN.

GENERAL VIEW

OF THE

AGRICULTURE

OF THE

COUNTY OF NAIRN,

THE

EASTERN COAST OF INVERNESS-SHIRE,

AND THE

PARISH OF DYKE, AND PART OF EDENKEILLIE,

IN THE

COUNTY OF ELGIN, AND FORRES.

BY JAMES DONALDSON,

FACTOR FOR THE HON WILLIAM RAMSAY MAULE, OF PANMURE

DRAWN UP FOR THE CONSIDERATION OF
THE BOARD OF AGRICULTURE AND INTERNAL IMPROVEMENT

LONDON
PRINTED BY B. MILLAN,
PRINTER TO HIS ROYAL HIGHNESS THE PRINCE OF WALES
M DCC.XCIV

TO THE READER.

IT is requested that this paper may be returned to the Board of Agriculture, at its Office in London, with any additional Remarks and Observations which may occur on the perusal, written on the Margin, as soon as may be convenient

It is hardly necessary to add, that this Report is, at present, printed and circulated for the purpose merely of procuring farther information respecting the Husbandry of this District, and of enabling every one to contribute his mite to the improvement of the country

The Board has adopted the same plan in regard to all the other Counties in the United Kingdom, and will be happy to give every assistance in its power, to any person who may be desirous of improving his breed of Cattle, Sheep, &c or of trying any useful Experiment in Husbandry

London, March 1794

COUNTY OF NAIRN, &c

INTRODUCTION

THE tract of country proposed to be described, lying towards the 58° of N latitude, comprehends the parish of Dyke, and part of Edenkeillie, in the county of Moray, the whole of the county of Nairn, and the eastern coast of Inverness-shire, to the mouth of the river Beaulie, from whence the extent along the Moray Frith, its northern boundary to the river Findhorn, is forty English miles   The county of Nairn stretches from the coast southerly to Lochindorb, about twenty miles, where it terminates nearly in a point between the counties of Elgin and Inverness   Its breadth along the shore is twelve miles, its sides extend to twenty two miles about the middle, from whence they begin to approximate each other   Exclusive of the hilly part of the district, it may be described as a narrow border of level ground along the shore, from one to nearly six miles in breadth

RIVERS.

1st, The river Beaulie, issuing from Loch Monar, in the western hills of Ross-shire, terminates the Moray Frith at Lovat, after a course of nearly sixty miles

2d, The river Ness   Descriptions of the course of this river are already before the public*, and the practicability of opening a communication to the Western Ocean, at Fort William, by joining Loch Ness to Loch Eoich, and that to Loch Lochy, and thence to the sea, has been satisfactorily establish-

---

* By Dr Anderson, and others

ed therefore it is only necessary to notice here, that this river forms the harbour at the town of Inverness

3d, The water of Nairn takes its rise in the hills of Inverness-shire, and after a course of nearly thirty miles, falls into the Frith at the town of Nairn. It is of little consequence, forming no harbour, and for salmon fishings yielding only a rent of about 8ol sterling.

SOIL AND CLIMATE

The soil of this district, lying under a climate almost as favourable as any in the kingdom, appears to be of three qualities. From the river Findhorn to the water of Nairn, comprehending the parishes of Dyke and Auldearn, the soil is a rich free loam generally on a sandy or gravelly bottom.

From Nairn to Inverness, comprehending the parishes of Nairn, Ardersier, Cawder, Croy, Petty, and part of Inverness, it is a light sandy soil; and from the river Ness to Beauly, including the low part of the parish of Inverness, and the part of Kirk-hill, the soil is either a stiff rich clay, or a sharp gravelly mould.

In the hilly part of the county of Nairn, the arable land is but in a small proportion to the waste, the soil is a sandy loam, full of gravel and small stones, except on the banks of the brooks, where it appears less mixed. In this quarter the climate is more cold and stormy than on the coast, and the productions of the soil are somewhat later. Yet the crops are never cut off by frost, nor is the harvest greatly more retarded by the autumnal rains than that of their neighbours in the more favourable situations.

There is a curious singularity connected with the soil of this district, namely, the sand which has nearly overwhelmed the estate of Cuvson, and which happened one time prior to the act of Parliament 1695, cap. 30, the narrative of which bears,

bears, " That the barony of Cowbin, and house and yards thereof, is quite ruined, and overspread with sand "

It appears that the sand washed up for ages by the tide on the coast towards the western limits of the parish of Dyke, was at last drifted by a storm of wind from the west, over the estate, one farm of which, now rented at about 80l alone remains, from which the land-tax and other public exactions are paid for an estate rated at nearly 1000l Scots, of valued rent, and which at present would probably, but for this accident, have rented at 800l sterling a year, or upwards

The extent of this calamity is not limited to the barony of Cowbin, it changed the efflux of the river Findhorn, by which a part of the estate of Maurton was destroyed, and drifting eastward for more than ten miles, buried a great extent of fine land in the parish of Duffus   But although this evil has not been felt on the east side of the river Findhorn during the present generation, yet its consequences are in a high degree to be feared   Besides the large extent of plain which it occupies, to the height, it is supposed, of the fruit-trees in the garden of Cowbin, a vast body is accumulated in a ridge of hills, called the hills of Mavistone, of strikingly conspicuous magnitude, these hills are observed to be gradually progressive, the sand drifting from the west, and settling on the lee of the east end   And there is reason to believe, that during the course of the last forty or fifty years, it has advanced eastward more than 100 yards.

Besides extending and promoting the growth of bent, a vegetable so peculiar to this soil, the landlords who are exposed to this dreadful visitation might certainly adopt some plan for fixing the sand within its present bounds   But it is neglected by all concerned, as if its encroachments were not to be apprehended, or as if they were in no degree prejudicial

The periods of wheat seed time and harvest which commenced on a particular farm in the neighbourhood of Inver-

ness

ness for the last four years, as stated below, will shew the earliness of the season

Wheat seed commenced in	-	-	-	1790,	9th November	
-	-	-	-	1791,	4th November	
		-		1792,	1st September	
	-	-	1793,	19th October		
Oats and peas seed commenced in		1791,	2d March			
-	-	-	-	1792,	3d March	
-	-	-	-	1793,	20th February	
Barley commenced in	-	-	1791,	16th April		
-	-	-	-	1792,	10th April	
	-	-	-	1793,	26th April	
Harvest commenced on the same farm in		1790,	6th Sep	& finished	19th Oct
-	-	-	-	1791,	21th Aug	—	11th Oct
-	-	-	-	1792,	6th Aug	—	9th Oct
-	-	-	-	1793,	5th Sept	—	16th Oct

TOWNS, POPULATION, AND MANUFACTURES

In this district there are two royal burghs, Inverness and Nairn, situated at the distance of eighteen miles from each other. The population of the town of Inverness amounts to 5257, and that of Nairn to 1400; there are also three villages, Dyke, Auldearn, and Campbeltown, which may contain from 50 to 100 houses in each.

There is a thread manufactory at Inverness, from which, on an average of the last seven years, there has been exported in white and coloured threads, to the extent of 13,000 l. sterling yearly. There is also a canvas and sail-cloth manufactory established there, from whence is exported annually upwards of 500,000 yards.

There is another species of manufacture carried on to a considerable extent in this district, that of the spinning of yarn. The flax is sent here by the merchants in Aberdeen, Dundee, Glasgow and Paisley, and returned to them in yarn. There is also a considerable quantity of timber and merchant goods carried

carried in open boats along the coast, to Caithness and the Orkney islands

From the port of Inverness there is exported annually raw wool to the value of 500 l sterling, and skins or peltry to the amount of 1200 l, but these last articles are the produce of the counties of Inverness, Nairn, and Ross-shire, at large

Though there is a great quantity of grain annually exported from that extent of coast, under the jurisdiction of the custom-house of Inverness, yet the quantity exported from the district now under review is very inconsiderable, the grain that can be spared by the farmers being in general requisite for the maintenance of the inhabitants of the towns and villages, and of those of the more remote parts of the Highlands

In the town of Nairn, though pleasantly and commodiously situated on the banks of the river, near the shore of the Frith, and having the advantage of the great north road passing through it, there are no manufactures of any kind some of the respectable inhabitants of the town seem extremely anxious to introduce some manufactories, in order to give employment to the inhabitants, and were the proprietors of the county to give their aid, there is little doubt but this desirable object might be attained

To the nine parishes already mentioned, that only of Ard-clach, in the hilly part of the county of Nairn, remains to be added, and the whole population, exclusive of the troops occasionally resident in Fort George, amounts to a little above twenty thousand

---

STATE OF PROPERTY.

In this district there are six proprietors, having each from 1000 l to 2500 l sterling a year, and twelve more, having each from 200 l to 800 l a year, the remainder, including the burgh lands of Inverness and Nairn, is divided into small estates, under 200 l sterling a year, amounting in all to 16,000 l

sterling

erling of yearly rent, exclusive of the rent of the salmon
fishings of Beaulie, Ness, and Nairn, which amount to 1870l
sterling

LAND, RENT, AND TENOR OF LEASES.

Although the greater part of the proprietors reside in the
district, yet it is plain that very little attention on their part
has been bestowed in promoting the improvement of the lands
occupied by the tenants such of the heritors, however, as
reside on their estate, have carried the improvements of their
own farms as high as the generality of the kingdom

Mr Davidson of Cantray, has in every particular ex-
tended his attention in the most judicious and successful manner beyond his own farm, over the whole of his estate, which
he found, about twenty years ago, when he came to reside
there bleak, poor and sterile in the extreme but it has now
assumed an appearance of neatness and fertility superior to any
other in that part of the district

There is but a very small proportion of this country pos-
essed by the tenants under leases in writing, scarcely one-
tenth of the whole Some of the leases are of endurance for
seven years others for eleven years, and a few for two nineteen years, but the greatest number are for nineteen years
There is no rotation of croping laid down in the leases, nor
(with a very few exceptions) is there any provision made as
to draining, inclosing, or leaving the lands in good condition
at the end of the lease

The general run of the farms pay from 15l to 20l of
yearly rent, burdened however in many cases with services,
carriages, mill restrictions, and a variety of small exactions
in kind, called cumm. There are, however, a few farms
of from one to three hundred acres

Tenants

Tenants enter into possession of houses, gardens and natural
pasture, at the term of Whitsunday, and to the arable land
the ingathering of that year's crop

The rents are paid partly in money, in grain, and in oatmeal, the money rent is paid at Martinmas, after reaping the
crop and the victual in March or April thereafter   It should
be remarked here, that the tenants on some estates in this
district are obliged to pay their farm meal at the rate of nine
stone and a half, and sometimes ten stone for the boll, a practice it is believed, little known in any other part of the
kingdom

The average rent by the acre over the whole district, exclusive of the natural pasturage, may be estimated at 13s
from which, however, the lands about the burghs of Inverness and Nairn, and around the villages above-mentioned,
are to be excepted, where in some cases the rents have risen
from 2l to nearly 5l the acre

THE MODE OF MANAGEMENT, AND IMPROVE-
MENTS OF HUSBANDRY

Although the proprietors, and the few more opulent and
intelligent farmers, have introduced fallow, green crops, and
sown grass into their practice, yet no stated or regular rotation of croping is here followed, unless that ancient system
which seems to have been the general practice before the æra
of the Reformation, and which is still almost universally
practised here by the ordinary and inferior class of tenants,
should be accounted a regular rotation   Almost the whole of
this country being uninclosed, the tenants are still accommodated with natural pasturage for their cattle, either in the
downs along the shore, or in the moors towards the bottom
of the mountains   On this account a very small proportion
of the arable land is considered as requisite for the pasture of
the

the stock on the small farms, a part of which, almost on every farm, consists of a small flock of sheep   These are shut up in the house every night, the floor of which is from time to time thickly covered with a bed of turf or sand, so as to form a kind of compost dung-hill, equal in surface to the area of the house   and from two to about four feet in depth   Besides this, the dung afforded by the black cattle and horses is also formed into a compost dung-hill, of which about three-fourths is generally *pure sand*, the least earthy and of largest particle being universally preferred   Of these two there must be amassed in the course of the year such a quantity as is sufficient to spread over one fourth of the farm, which, after three ploughings, is generally sown with Scots bear, at the rate of four firlots to the acre, between the middle of May and the middle of June   And this, with the exception of a portion allowed for potatoes, and occasionally a small patch in flax, for domestic accommodation, is uniformly succeeded by two or three successive crops of oats, the oats sown between the first week of March and the last week of April, and after one ploughing, which is performed during the winter, or at the time of sowing, and four firlots of seed is allowed to the acre   and if the land, under this management, becomes so much over-run with weeds of different kinds as not to return double the seed, which is not unfrequently the case, it is allowed to lye waste for one or two years, during which it is pastured by the cows and horses, and again brought under cultivation, and treated in the same manner as above described

On the large farms, and on such lands as are occupied by the proprietors, and where fallow green crops and sown grass are introduced into the system, the most improved and judicious mode of managing the dung, and laying down the different crops, prevail

The system adopted by the generality of farmers, as above described, is the necessary result of their having no certain leases, and although, before the depreciation of the value of

money

money by its increased abundance in the present age, this system might have afforded the comforts of life suited to the ideas of the times, yet it is a system which at the present day uniformly condemns its followers to all the evils of poverty, and consequently prevents them from possessing the means or the inclination for improvement

This becomes conspicuous by the mere inspection only of their extremely imperfect implements of agriculture, which, with very few exceptions, are fabricated by the tenants themselves It is unnecessary to describe the clumsy aukwardness of the plough, in the construction of which there is comparatively very little iron employed The carts are framed on a form still further from perfection the wheels, about two feet diameter, are composed only of three pieces of plank two or three inches hick, having square holes in the centre to receive the axle, which must therefore turn round with the wheels, moving in wooden bows fixed under the body of the cart The shafts are formed of the larger, and the body of the carriage of bars or slender batons of the smaller branches of the alder tree It not being intended to recommend this model for imitation, it is needless to describe the straw collar, the saddle, or the timber crupper, or to calculate the inferiority of the power of the horses in such contemptible harness, or the difference between the load which is drawn and that which might be drawn by the same horses in a cart and harness of more perfect construction

It is only further necessary to mention the kellach sledge, a conical basket framed of twigs, supported with its base uppermost between the shafts and two cross bars, by which the shafts are connected, which is still commonly used, and which is sometimes drawn without wheels of any kind.

On the farms of the proprietors, and on the large farms, ploughs, carts, harrows, and every other implement employed in the field, are constructed on the best principles, and in the most perfect manner

LABOUR-

LABOURERS, AND THE EXPENCE OF LABOUR

Though there are no manufactures in this district, besides those already mentioned, yet the price of labour has nearly doubled in the course of the last twenty years this perhaps may be accounted for by the great number of both sexes in that class going to the south of Scotland, in order to procure work in summer and harvest, from whence they return with such a stock of money in their pockets, as enables them to spend the winter with some degree of comfort

The wages of an ordinary ploughman, exclusive of bed and board, are from 5l to 6l sterling a year, and those of a female servant from 1l 15s to 2l 5s labourers by the day have even-pence or eight-pence and their victuals

A man engaged for the harvest, which generally lasts six weeks, receive 1l and a woman from 14s to 17s

The farm servants, with few exceptions, lodge and eat in the family they are maintained nearly in the same manner though at a much less expence, than those in the county of Moray, as was more fully described in the report of that district Potatoes, and the small herrings which are caught in great quantities in the Frith, supply a great proportion of the food of the poorer people, servants and labourers

———

ROADS AND BRIDGES

In the report of the county of Moray, the convenience, practicability and expence of erecting a bridge across the river Findhorn, was pretty fully detailed, it is only further necessary here to add, that if this interesting improvement were by any means obtained, the course of the post-road through this district could be conducted in a line much more advantageous to the inhabitants and to the public at large, and it is humbly suggested, that the best possible direction, both in regard to a

proper

proper level, and to every other object which ought to be attended to in a work of this kind, would be to carry this road from the proposed bridge to be built across the Findhorn, by the north side of the Earl of MORAY's plantations at Darnway, along the south side of the moss of Litie, through the lands of Auldearn, and from thence to the bridge over the water of Nairn, on the military road to Fort George, from thence through the inclosures of Kilravock, holding westward to the church of Croy, until it meet the present highway about a mile farther west

There are several advantages which would be gained by this direction of the road the rivulet called the burn of Daltey, could never impede the traveller so near its source as Earl's Mill, where at any rate a bridge could be afforded from the public funds of the county

But what would be of much more advantage to the inhabitants of the country, is, that this direction of the post road would open up an immediate and direct communication through the most valuable tract of arable land in the district the advantages of this need not be pointed out, even to any farmer of ordinary observation, or of common understanding, yet from these obvious advantages this part of the country is entirely debarred by the present course of the post road, which i directed on the outside of the country, and excepting part of the parish of Dyke, and the town of Nairn, it is conducted along the most sterile and the most thinly inhabited tract in the low part of the district

The direction of the road here pointed out, would open to all the country an easy and ready access to an almost inexhaustible fund of rich pure marl, which has been hitherto locked up in the moss of Litie, and another quarter of the country would be hereby also equally enriched, by a similar access to the marl pits lately opened at Kinstarie

The military road from Strathspey to Fort George, by Dalsy bridge, has been lately completed in the most masterly

c   manner,

manner, insomuch that it is not easy to form an idea that there is any thing further required for its improvement, and much credit is certainly due to those under whose directions this work was planned and executed

The other roads were made and repaired under the authority of the Act of Parliament 1669 of them it is only necessary to observe, that they merit no commendation, and that they remain susceptible of great improvements, which might certainly be effected even under this Act of Parliament, if proper attention was paid by those who are charged with the execution of this branch of police

The landholders in Inverness-shire have lately applied for and obtained an Act of Parliament, for levying conversion money in lieu of labour, and for making and repairing highways and bridges in that shire, by which means it is to be hoped both the public and parochial roads will in a few years be put in a proper state of repair

MARKETS AND FAIRS.

In the towns of Inverness and Nairn there are regular weekly markets, where butcher meat, meal, butter, cheese, poultry, eggs, and such articles, are sold, and where also considerable quantities of fuel is brought for sale by the poorer tenants in the neighbourhood, and from the sale of such articles these tenants are on the other hand supplied with salt, and such other articles as they consider necessary, and by this means also, a part of their money rent is scraped together

Butcher meat and fish, though still moderate compared to the prices in other parts of the kingdom, have, notwithstanding, of late years advanced very considerably in this district

Butcher meat sells at from 2d to 3d the pound, haddocks from 6d to 1s the dozen, poultry 6d each, ducks 7d or 8d geese from 1s 6d to 2s and turkeys 3s each, eggs about 2d the dozen

The

The average price of grain and oatmeal for the last seven years, will be seen by the annexed fiars of the county of Inverness and Nairn

FIARS OF INVERNESS SHIRE FOR THE CROPS 1786 AND 1792, AND THE INTERMEDIATE CROPS AND YEARS

Years	Wheat			Bear			Pease			Oats & Oatmeal		
	£	s	d	£	s	d	£	s	d	£	s	d
1786	1	0	0	0	17	0	0	15	0	0	15	0
1787	1	0	0	0	17	0	0	15	0	0	15	0
1788	1	4	0	0	15	6	0	13	4	0	13	4
1789	1	1	0	0	16	0	0	13	6	0	13	6
1790	1	1	0	0	17	0	0	15	6	0	15	6
1791	0	19	0	0	18	0	0	16	0	0	16	0
1792	1	0	0	0	18	0	0	15	0	0	15	0

FIARS OF NAIRN-SHIRE FOR THE CROPS 1786 AND 1792, AND THE INTERMEDIATE CROPS AND YEARS

Years	Wheat			Barley			Oats			Oatmeal			Pease			Bear			Rye		
	£	s	d	£	s	d	£	s	d	£	s	d	£	s	d	£	s	d	£	s	d
1786	1	1	0	0	17	0	0	15	0	0	15	0	0	15	0	0	15	0	0	15	0
1787	1	0	0	0	17	0	0	16	0	0	15	0	0	15	0	0	15	0	0	15	0
1788	1	4	0	0	14	6	0	13	6	0	13	0	0	13	0	0	13	0	0	13	0
1789	1	1	0	0	15	0	0	13	6	0	13	0	0	13	0	0	13	0	0	13	0
1790	1	0	0	0	16	0	0	15	6	0	15	0	0	15	0	0	15	0	0	15	0
1791	1	0	0	0	18	0	0	18	0	0	16	0	0	16	0	0	16	0	0	16	0
1792	1	0	0	0	17	0	0	14	0	0	14	0	0	14	0	0	14	0	0	14	0

In Inverness there are seven fairs during the course of the year, in which black cattle, horses, sheep, implements of husbandry, and country commodities, are sold. At these fairs the country people from the remotest parts of the North and West Highlands are in the practice of providing themselves with those articles which they must necessarily have, and which is generally done by the barter of their butter, cheese, peltry, and such other merchandize as their situation enable them to bring to market.

In the town of Nairn there are also six stated fairs in the year, in which business similar to that of Inverness fairs is negotiated to a certain extent. But as Inverness lyes on the one side, and Forres on the other, and both better situated for a trade of this kind, the stated fairs which are held in the town of Nairn are comparatively of little consequence, as the inhabitants of a small corner of the country only attend them.

FARM HOUSES AND OFFICES

The few farmers who possess what are here considered as extensive farms, are well accommodated with houses. They are built in a substantial manner, of stone and lime, and either slated, or thatched with straw; they appear sufficiently commodious and properly situated; but it must be observed, that they are in general built at the tenant's expence. He is obliged to lay out the money in the first instance, and the proprietor is only bound by the lease to allow him a certain proportion of the expence at his removal. If the value of the houses should exceed the sum stipulated in the lease, by the custom of the country, it is left optional to the tenant either to carry off the surplus value, or to bargain with his successor on such terms as they may agree upon, or as two men to be mutually chosen by them, may determine.

The habitations of the poorer tenants in the district, however, are mean, dark and dirty cottages built of turf, without
order

order or connexion with each other   The proprietor in general affords what is called the great timber, and the tenant is
at the expence of cutting the turf and erecting the fabric   The
district is by no means destitute of stone, and therefore, by a
little expence and attention on the part of the proprietors, and
of those who have the management of their estates, this class
of people might be accommodated with lodgings much warmer
and more healthy than those in which they are at present
obliged to reside

In the villages above-mentioned, the houses are in general
built of stone, and slated, or properly thatched either with
straw, or with bent from the downs along the shore

LIVE STOCK.

It will be naturally inferred from the preceding account of
the state of the country, and from the system of husbandry
generally practised, that there is but little attention paid to the
improvement of stock, and that they must be comparatively
of little value

Black Cattle—Agreeable to the ancient practice, which
was taken notice of in the agricultural report of Moray, oxen
are still for the most part employed in the plough on the ordinary sized farms, and when the seed season is over, towards
the end of June, they are generally boarded for about three
months, at the rate of from 1s 3d to 1s 6d each, in the glens
and mountains in the Highlands   Their pile, by this management, is no doubt much improved, but the labour requisite to procure their food, and the cold to which they are
exposed, is not very favourable to the other qualifications
which are regarded in the species, yet the breed remains un-
mixed, neither crossed with the Lancashire or Dutch, and
exhibit when in flesh, a more handsome figure than the herds
of the county of Moray   They are, however, of a smaller
bone,

bone, weighing when fat only from 18 to 24 stone, Amsterdam. The number in this district amounts to upwards of 11,000 and when three years old, the general value may be estimated at from 2l. 15s. to 3l. each.

Horses.—In this report it is unnecessary to take notice of the farm horses belonging to the proprietors and the more opulent farmers, because they are nearly equal in height and value to the horses in other parts of the kingdom where two horse ploughs have been introduced.

The horses which are reared by the most attentive farmers in the middling and lower classes, are generally from seven to nine hands high, and when five or six years old, they sell at from 7l. to 10l. sterling. There are, however, a number of horses in the district, which do not sell when in their prime for much above the half of these prices. The number of horses of all kinds in the district is nearly 4000, and the average price when five years old, may be from 7l. to 8l.

Sheep.—It has been observed, that a certain number of this species of stock is to be seen on all the small farms. They are almost without exception of the small white faced kind and appear to be the original breed of the country. A score of wedders taken from the flock, without particular selection in regard to size, sell, about the end of harvest, when fattest, at from 6l. to 7l. the score, at which season such wedders weigh from six to eight pounds the quarter. The wool is for the most part manufactured in the family, for bed-clothes and apparel. When sold at Inverness or Nairn, the price is about 8s. the stone. The whole number is about 18,500, and the medium price may be about five shillings.

DRAINS.

From the preceding description of the soil of this district, it will be understood that the arable lands are in general dry

In

In the country called the *Aird*, of which the parish of Kirk-hill is a part, where the soil is a deep rich clay, open drains properly constructed would be a great improvement, as appears from the good effects of those already made

In this district there are several small lakes, some consisting of marshy, and others of mossy ground, that might be easily cleared of water, yet in general the inducement to lay out the requisite expence must be the expectation of finding marl, rather than making any addition to the corn fields. In the parish of Kirk-hill, however, a considerable acquisition of arable land might be gained at a small expence, by draining the lake, or loch of Conan   Another improvement of more consequence might be effected, and a great extent of the most valuable land in the district brought into a state of cultivation, were an embankment to be formed along the shore of the Frith, from the mouth of the river Beaulie to the estate of Warrandfield, so as to secure this extensive tract, consisting of several hundred acres, from being overflowed or injured by the Moray Frith   One gentleman, Major FRASER of Belladrum, who rents a farm here from the Hon Mr FRASER of Lovat, the proprietor of all these grounds along the shore, has done a great deal in order to secure his farm, and has thereby evinced the practicability of converting the whole of this plain, the greatest part of which is now in a state of nature, into rich arable corn fields   It is to be hoped the proprietor will study his own interest, and that of the country at large, by following out the plan so judiciously and so successfully begun by Major FRASER

But an improvement of still greater consequence, and more extensively useful to the country, might be made at an expence comparatively small, were Mr CAMPBELL of Calder to drain the moss of Litle, in which, it is already ascertained, there is an almost inexhaustible stock of rich pure marl. Those only who are acquainted with the improvements which have been effected in Strathmore, and in other parts of the county of Angus, by the use of this valuable manure, can form any judgment of the advantages which must necessarily result to this gentleman and to the neighbouring proprietors, were this moss drained, and marl brought into general use as a manure. Except on the estate of Cantray, there are no lime quarries in the district, and the expence of importing lime from the Frith of Forth, or the north of England, amounts almost to a prohibition, at least insomuch that there is little chance of this species of manure ever coming into general use in this district. On that account therefore, the opening of this store of marl becomes an object of still greater importance. As an inducement to Mr CAMPBELL to execute this important work, it may not be improper here to state, that a gentleman in Angus, Mr DEMPSTER of Dunichen, whose spirited exertions to promote the good of his country are so well known as to require no commentary here, a few years ago drained a lake on his estate in which marl had been discovered, and the last year cleared upwards of 900l. sterling after paying all expences.

There is indeed just now some thousand bolls of very good marl lying ready for market on Mr GORDON's estate of Kinstarie, but even the most intelligent tenants in that neighbourhood seem totally ignorant of the value of this new discovered treasure, and have not yet had resolution to make one single experiment of its effects, even though sufficient proofs have been afforded them, by the greatest crops of corn, grass and turnips produced thereby on Mr GORDON's own farm. It is however certain, that both these gentlemen, as well as the other proprietors in the neighbourhood, have it in their power, by the leases which they grant in future, of obliging their tenants to use marl as a manure, and if this is done, under proper regulations (which ought to be very carefully attended to, and which will probably be detailed in the report of the county of Ayr) it is evident that it is the best security they can have for the improvement of their estates, and the punctual payment of their rents.

WOODS

WOODS AND PLANTATIONS.

Although this district is by no means destitute of wood, yet its general appearance, except for two or three miles west of the river Findhorn, and about Inverness, seems bleak and naked, and as the plantations are in general situated in the higher parts of the country, it is evident they afford no shelter to the arable lands It would certainly add much to the beauty of the country, as well as improvement in regard to climate, were the proprietors to plant the rising grounds which are intermixed with the corn fields, but inaccessible to the plough Of such there are a great many all over the country, particularly on the estates of Culloden, Castle Stewart, and Kinstarie The proprietors of the parish of Inverness have adopted this plan, and if they proceed for a few years, it is probable there will not be a single useless acre in that parish It must be observed also, that every proprietor's family seat in the district is ornamented with plantations, containing every species of forest trees

Extensive plantations, though principally of Scots fir, are to be seen on almost every estate in the higher part of the country, and on some of the moors in the low country, and Mr DAVIDSON of Cantray has within these twenty years planted upwards of two thousand acres The country at present not only supplies itself, but also a considerable part of the adjoining county of Elgin and Forres, with timber for the ordinary implements of husbandry, and for the buildings and furniture of the country people, and there is no doubt but in a few years the export of timber from this district will be an article of considerable value

It would be improper in a report of this kind, not to take particular notice of the Earl of MORAY's extensive forests on his estate of Darnway, and of those also on his Lordship's estate of Castle Stewart

These are of very great extent, covering upwards of 3600 Scots acres, all within the district under review Of this

extent

extent the greatest part lyes in the parish of Edenkellie, and part in that of Dyke, stretching along the banks of the Find- horn and forming an immense circle round the ancient Castle of Darnwa. The remainder, about 600 acres, lyes in the parish of Petty, near to Castle Stewart. They were begun by the present Earl in the year 1767. The Scots fir is used for nursing up and sheltering the more valuable kinds of deci- duous trees, of which the oak is the principal object of atten- tion. These are planted among the firs at the distances at which they are intended to stand when full grown, and as soon as the firs have performed this office, they are to be al- together taken away, so that the whole will form a noble forest of oaks intermixed with the other valuable deciduous trees. In some of the older plantations the firs are already completely cut out, and exhibit forest scenes vastly superior to that of the gloomy Scots fir so frequent in Scotland. Every attention has been paid to the preservation and proper thinning of these plantations, and the natural consequence has been, that they have throve extremely, many of them, about nine- teen years old, measuring about twenty inches in girth at three feet from the ground. The firs are planted out at two years old from the seed bed, and when of size sufficient to afford proper shelter, pits are made amongst them, into which the oaks and other trees are planted, often standing two years in the seed bed, and three or four years in the nursery. To shew with what spirit these plantations have been carried on, it may be proper to mention, that in one season, viz between Autumn 1782 and Summer 1783, no fewer than 75,000 oaks were planted out. From the failure in England of the acorn crop sometimes for two or three seasons following, it is impossible to make the progress which could be wished, in filling up these extensive plantations with oaks, as all the young plants are raised in the Earl's own gardens at Darnway. An exact register being kept of all the trees annually planted out, a copy of the amount of each class has been obtained, which is here subjoined.

Oaks

Oaks planted between November 1767 and Summer 1793 - - -	614,500
Ash, beech, elm, sycamore, Spanish chesnut, spruce firs and larix, during same period	336,500
Scots firs betwixt November 1767 and Summer 1787 - - - -	9,687,000
Total	10,638,000

A period of many years will be requisite for filling up these extensive plantations with oaks, but the work is going regularly forward

The thinnings of the firs are sold from two-pence to four-pence per dozen but the demand of the country is not equal to the quantities necessarily taken out A few years ago a part of them were carried by sea to Newcastle and Sunderland, for the use of the coal-works in that neighbourhood

On the opposite banks of the Findhorn a similar mode of planting has been followed by Mr CUMIN of Nelugas, and since 1779 above two hundred acres have been covered, and about 80,000 oaks planted out

MISCELLANEOUS OBSERVATIONS,

AND

HINTS FOR IMPROVEMENT

The means of improvement have been hinted at in general, or may be inferred from the state of the country as already described. It is obvious that this district is in general more backward in the state of agriculture, and in the condition of the common people, than their neighbours to the southward It is also obvious, that the arable land, by judicious management, might be rendered greatly more productive, and that the value of the cattle, horses and sheep, might be increased many-fold

It

It s however not to be supposed, that any lasting and general improvement can be on a sudden, or all at once, introduced into any country, even although the landlords were to bestow their united and best directed efforts for that purpose It must be many years before the land, under the management of the country people can be brought into the most improved condition of which it s susceptible   The proprietor however, ought not to be discouraged, for it is evident that they may in a few years, by proper attention, bring about a surprising alteration in the state of things, and in the appearance of the country   In order to effectuate this, it appears necessary to enlarge the farms to an extent sufficient for the employment of a reasonable capital, which should be applied in the cultivation of the farm only, without being directed to other purposes, such as building houses, or inclosing the farm, the expence of which should be advanced by the proprietor, on a moderate interest to be paid by the tenant.

One objection only can be stated against the propriety of enlarging the farms, and that is the removing the present set of tenants, but this certainly might be obviated, were the proprietors to feu out some detached corners of their estates properly situated in regard to fuel and water, and introduce some manufactures to give employment to the people   They would in that case live much more comfortably than they do at present, and at the same time become more useful members of the state   It may be unnecessary to repeat, that no spirited cultivation of land can be performed by the poor inhabitants of a dark damp smoaky hovel, when it is further considered that the labouring cattle are still more wretchedly accommodated

The want of leases must be an insurmountable bar to improvements in agriculture

In countries highly cultivated, where the inclosures are completed, and regular rotations of croping introduced, a lease of nineteen years is considered both by proprietor and tenant as a reasonable period, but in such a country as this, where so much rests with the tenant to perform, it might be highly proper to add eight or ten years more to this duration, so that the tenant may be satisfied he can reap the fruits of his own labour, skill and improvements, without the fear of being turned out by another

From the consideration that all people are extremely reluctant to quit old habits, and to venture on untried experiments, perhaps it might be proper that the first leases which are granted, should oblige the holders to have a certain proportion of the farm in fallow, clover, and turnip

Were regular rotations of croping to be adopted, the following appears likely to turn out the most advantageous for that part of the district from Findhorn to Inverness

First year---Turnip, land dunged.

Second year---Barley, with 8 lb white and 8 lb red clover, 4 lb rib-grass, and one and a half or two bushels of rye-grass.

Third year---Grass to be made into hay

Fourth year---Grass to be pastured

Fifth year---Grass to be pastured

Sixth year---Grass to be pastured

Seventh year---Oats

Eighth year---Barley

In the low part of the parish of Kirk-hill, where the soil and climate are nearly equal to that of the Carse of Gowrie, the same rotation of croping which after many years experience is now considered the most advantageous there, might be introduced into this part of the district with great propriety, and is as follows

First year---Fallow, the land dunged

Second year---Wheat

Third year---Pease or beans

Fourth year---Barley, with 20 lb red clover, and one bushel rye-grass

Fifth year---Grass

Sixth year---Oats

But

But no regular rotation of croping can be adopted in any country, unless the fields are laid out in proper order, and where pasture grass makes part of the system, it is absolutely necessary that the farm should be inclosed, and subdivided In this country in general, that can only be done by thorn hedges, as more fences could only be erected on particular estates where quarries abound From every information that could be procured, there is reason to believe, that were the proprietors to grant leases for twenty one or twenty seven years many of the tenants would chearfully concur with them in bearing a proportion of the expence of rearing and protecting hedges, and also agree to pay interest for the money expended in making these inclosures

Besides the other advantages of inclosing, which are so well known that they need not be here pointed out, it is certain that the breed of stock would be thereby greatly improved It has been long supposed, that the cattle raised on the inclosed farms in the occupation of the proprietors, are of a superior breed to those raised by the tenants in the adjoining open fields, because they are so greatly superior in weight and figure, but all this superiority is nothing more than the result of the ease, shelter, freedom, and more plentiful food with which they are supplied in these inclosures, accordingly it is found, that the small cattle raised by the poorest people in the district, when pastured but a few years in the meadows of England, attain near double their former size

It is needless to resume the reflections on the mill restrictions, services and customs, or on the carriages and other labour exacted by the landlords The experience of the whole landlords in the highest improved counties of Scotland, have demonstrated how much the annual returns of an estate are increased by abolishing every species of personal thraldom

Although the sands of Cowbin, from the familiarity of the scene, may be disregarded by those in that vicinity, yet to every attentive strnager it exhibits a most singular landscape,
and

and while it recalls his idea of the past, it also excites appre-
hensions respecting its future encroachments The Act of
Parliament for the preservation of bent has proved an ineffec-
tual check, as it is now currently pulled, and sold for thatch-
ing the houses in the country, and that with the tacit appro-
bation at least of those proprietors whose interests are most
deeply concerned Planting broad belts of the quickest grow-
ing trees on the nearest uncovered ground, appears to be the
most certain barrier that can be obtained, and this ground
being in general deep and moist, would be favourable to the
growth of such trees

From the preceding report it will appear, that except the
lands occupied by the proprietors, and by some few intelligent and respectable farmers, no improvements have taken
place in the cultivation of the arable lands, yet still it is per-
fectly evident that the country is very capable of the highest
cultivation, and though it is not probable, as has been
already observed, that any general improvement can be established all at once, yet it is certain that the proprietors, and
those in the management of their estates, have it much in
their power gradually to introduce better modes of husbandry,
which, it is humbly supposed, can best be effected by enlarging the size of the farms, granting leases of proper duration,
adopting regular rotations of croping, inclosing the lands, and
building proper farm houses, without obliging the tenant to
expend any part of his stock in procuring the necessary accommodation in these respects -

There are two gentlemen, Mr FORBES of Culloden, and
Mr GORDON of Kiustarie, who are about to grant leases
over their estates in this district From their public spirit it
is to be expected that they will not miss so favourable an op-
portunity of introducing a regular system of husbandry on
their estates, which would not only secure the complete improvement of them, but also promote the general interests of
the country, for unless some public spirited proprietors will

make

make such arrangements on their estates, and use some such measures as where pointed out, the country must long remain in its present unimproved state, and it cannot be supposed that the present set of tenants considering the circumstances in which they are placed, will ever adopt any spirited plan for the improvement of the country or of their own situation

FORT GEORGE

This Fort is situated on the point of Airderseer, near the middle of the northern boundary of this district Government once proposed to build it at Inverness, at a place called the Crown or Cromwell's Fort, but the magistrates of Inverness demanded such a price for the ground, that the Duke of CUMBERLAND was offended, and ordered an inspection of the ground whereon it now stands to be made by some engineers who reported that it would answer equally well with that at Inverness Accordingly Government purchased the ground, and a large farm in the neighbourhood of it, from Mr CAMPBELL of Calder The works commenced in the year 1747 under the direction of General SKINNER The estimate given in was 120,000l but it is said to have cost upwards of 160,000l It is a most regular fortification, and is the only one built in Britain according to a regular plan It covers ten Scots acres It does not appear to have had any considerable influence on the state of society in the country around, the market, however, which it has opened for several productions of the country, renders it an object of some consideration in an agricultural view It might therefore be improper to conclude this report without taking some notice of this superb and expensive establishment

THE END

Lightning Source UK Ltd.
Milton Keynes UK
UKHW051922240822
407764UK00006B/658